Clean

The only real way to be naturally skinny, lose weight, and have more energy than you can possibly imagine

Table of Contents

INTRODUCTION 1

CHAPTER 1: WHAT IS "EATING CLEAN"? 3

CHAPTER 2: WHY JOIN THE CLEAN EATING MOVEMENT? 7

CHAPTER 3: HOW TO CLEAN UP YOUR EATING 11

CHAPTER 4: EATING CLEAN ON A BUDGET 17

CHAPTER 5: EATING CLEAN ON THE GO 23

CHAPTER 6: EATING CLEAN FOR WEIGHT LOSS 27

CONCLUSION 33A

Your Free Bonus: Get this FREE Report

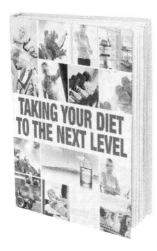

As a thank you, I want to give you this amazing report entitled **Taking Your Diet to the Next Level**, completely free of charge, as my gift to you. Download it now!

Click here to get it FREE!!

http://bit.ly/nextleveldiet

Introduction

I want to thank you and congratulate you for downloading the book, Clean Eating.

This book contains proven steps and strategies on how and why to change your lifestyle to cleaner and healthier eating without feeling deprived or breaking your budget.

In this book, you'll find out what clean eating really means and how to incorporate it into your daily life. You'll also discover the broader implications that eating clean has for both our environment and our personal health, along with tips for eating clean on a budget, on-the-go, and for losing weight.

Thanks again for downloading this book, I hope you enjoy it!

Chapter 1: What is "eating clean"?

Move over Mediterranean, Paleo, South Beach, and Atkins! The latest diet buzzword is "eating clean". Touted by gorgeous celebrities, such as Nicole Kidman and Jessica Alba, as the solution to that "nagging baby weight" and a cure for most other ills, it can be a little confusing what they're actually talking about. What are they eating...or not eating? How do they make it "clean"? And, is it like that salmon and caviar diet thing that no real person could ever afford to do?

Actually clean eating is a concept that's been around for a long time, spreading slowly but relentlessly. It's more of a lifestyle than a diet, and you may already be eating cleaner than you know. In the 1990's, there was a groundswell movement against chemical substances in food, particularly artificial sweeteners. Many had been shown to be carcinogens, and people began to avoid buying products containing the worst culprits. The average Joe had started to read the labels and wasn't thrilled with what he found there! In an effort to "clean up" their products, supermarkets began to revise ingredient lists, particularly on store brands, by removing items that were unrecognizable as "food". This was actually a controversial move on their part, since it could mean removing added nutrients (that had been listed by their technical names) and also the loss of some relatively harmless but universally desirable preservatives. These pitfalls were avoided by listing nutrients by their common names (pantothenic acid = a B vitamin) and by clearly identifying preservatives as such on labels. The "clean eating" movement had truly begun.

Health food stores started doing better business than ever before; soon organic supermarkets, like Whole Foods and Trader Joe's, began to proliferate across the land; growing your own vegetables and shopping at farmer's markets were on the upswing; then, organic produce and products crept quietly into your local supermarket, and "farm to table" became the new buzzword for restaurants. Next came the question of the safety of genetically modified organisms [GMO's] that you may have read about and which is still being debated. It's all part of the growing concern on the part of average consumers with exactly what was and is going into their bodies. And, it's the history of "eating clean".

Clean eating is not a diet *per se*, but rather a concept: eating natural unprocessed foods is the best thing for you. Not raw, mind you, but *unprocessed*. Foods with nothing taken away, yes, but also foods with nothing added. You don't need to harvest your own rice from a paddy in your back yard; it's OK if it comes in a bag or a box as long as it's unrefined and has only one ingredient, rice. Apply that to everything you eat, and you're eating clean, my friend! Replace pre-packaged foods with the homemade versions. Use only fresh local produce. It sounds simple---and it *is* a simple idea. Think of it as "retro" style eating, like our forefathers (and foremothers) ate. Clean healthy natural food! Great! Sure!

So, what's the catch? That's also simple. Most of us lead very different lives from those healthy-eating ancestors of ours. We don't live on the land, keep our own chickens, or grow oats on the lower forty acres. Who has time to kill and pluck a chicken before turning it into nuggets to feed to the kids (who also have much busier lives), even on the weekend? Many of us don't have the space, time, inclination, or ability to grow our own food, and running all over town to get fresh food is time-consuming and can get very expensive. Is eating clean only for wealthy celebrities or backwoods hillbillies then? Really, why should I bother? Read on!

Chapter 2: Why join the clean eating movement?

We'll set aside for right now <u>how</u> you can eat clean without mega-bucks and still maintain a normal life. First let's talk about WHY you should. There are numerous personal benefits to eating clean, as well as long-term environmental issues that become entangled in the equation. What you eat is more important in many more than ways than you thought!

Food provides the basic foundation of every cell in your body and also supplies the materials for their continuing maintenance and repair. It's like preventative medicine, but more tasty. It keeps you functioning well and strengthens your immune system. You've heard the expression "Garbage in, garbage out". It's as true for your body as it is for computers! Quality maintenance requires quality materials. You know this; it's why you don't put junky used oil back in your car. Why do less for your body?

As people clean up their eating, they report numerous health benefits. Those of you who have cut back or even eliminated your intake of some "big baddies" will know what I mean. Salt and sugar are actually addictive substances---the more you eat, the more you want, and the less you taste how much is there. Cut them out of your diet, and your body lets you know it wants them back! Now! But suffer through the withdrawal and you feel different on the other side. You notice changes in digestion, sleep, and mood. Good changes! Clean eating eliminates far more alien substances from your system than simply lowering your sugar intake does, and its effect is much more far-reaching.

The list of health benefits from eating clean is long and varied. People report clearer thinking, fewer aches and pains, better mood and sleep quality, more energy, and healthier skin and hair. Clean eating is believed to help lower your risk of heart disease, stroke, and certain cancers. It's also useful in preventing anemia and osteoporosis. Bloating and fatigue go away and sex drive improves. Wow, has that got your attention? These changes won't happen overnight, but adherents of clean eating will tell you that it won't be very long before you notice the improvements to your overall health and well being. You'll feel better all over. You'll also notice the difference right away if, and when, you slip back into your old eating habits!

Clean eating has also been touted as a "diet" in the weight loss sense. This is where celebrities have spread the word and created the buzz. Several factors of eating clean are indeed very beneficial in losing weight. By increasing consumption of fresh fruits and vegetables and decreasing (or eliminating) processed foods, most people are automatically taking in fewer calories. They're also getting more fiber, which keeps them from feeling quite so hungry and makes it easier to continue eating less. Eating frequent small meals helps in boosting metabolism, increasing energy levels help get them moving more, and the higher intake of water keeps them hydrated. All of these work together to assist the body in shedding excess weight and keeping it off.

But the implications of eating clean go beyond personal health. Many of the things avoided by going "clean", such as man-made pesticides, meat treated with hormones and antibiotics, and artificial additives, colors, and preservatives, ultimately have an impact on our planet. Clean eating considers not only the effect of these items and issues on <u>you</u> but also their effect on the world around you, with direct bearing on the sustainability of our food supply. It questions how modern food production could be related to such global issues as antibiotic-resistant bacteria and the ocean's "dead zones". What's the effect of all these things on human health, metabolism, or the emotional and physical development of children? Could they have contributed to the drastic rise in childhood allergies or the increase in learning disabilities? What about cancer and diabetes? These are important issues, and they're what connect clean eating to a social and cultural movement that goes way beyond weight loss and shiny hair.

Chapter 3: How to clean up your eating

Becoming a clean eater doesn't need to happen all at once. It's just not an all-or-nothing proposition, not a sudden conversion. This is a lifestyle change that you can implement gradually. Many of you have probably already made changes in the foods you buy and eat because of an increased awareness of ingredients, and therefore you've "cleaned' some of your eating already. With a little thought and planning, you can eat even cleaner and help the planet, too. So let's talk about the basic tenets of clean eating before we discuss the implementation of them.

Eating clean is not really complicated or difficult to understand. There's no fancy measuring, no counting calories, no special beverages or weird combinations of food. It just involves doing a few simple things:

Avoiding food that:
- is processed or refined
- contains artificial ingredients
- is grown using chemical pesticides or fertilizers

- is raised with antibiotics or hormones

- Eating small meals 5-6 times a day

- Eating lean protein and complex carbs at each meal

- Drinking 2-3 quarts of water each day

- Eating local and in season whenever possible

The first hurdle is to shake the media hype that food companies have bombarded you with for so long. You need to read ingredients, not advertising. That's important so I'll repeat---**you need to read ingredients**. Phrases like zero trans-fat, reduced sugar, and low sodium are really meaningless. Reduced from what? Lowered from what? And how? Processing! These phrases and others are simply ways to make you believe that the particular processed food is healthier somehow. It's not---it's still processed. To eat clean you need to know what's **in** the food. So read the ingredients. Do you recognize these items? Are they pronounceable? Does it remind you of a recipe list? Then you've got "clean" food, even if it's boxed or bagged. Zealots will say, "Don't eat anything with more than five ingredients!" But you don't really need to go there, especially since that would eliminate homemade chocolate chip cookies too! If it sounds like real food, it's probably clean. Keep an eye out, however, for those sneaky words "enriched", "refined", and "processed" since they all indicate that the food has been treated or changed somehow. Once you start taking the time to read the labels, you'll automatically start making better choices at the store. After all, how tasty does "tertiary butylhydroquinone" sound? And, yes, that's a real ingredient found on food labels, sometimes shortened to TBHQ! Start reading; you'll find it!

What to do about chemical fertilizers and pesticides, hormones, and antibiotics? The simplest way is to go organic, although admittedly that can be pricey. If you buy local produce and meats, you're less likely to find that these items have been used. Of course, growing and hunting your own is another option for some. Locally grown or raised foods have also not been treated with preservatives to keep them fresh longer. That's why local grapes, for instance, are "cleaner" than out of season grapes that have been imported. Something has to keep them fresh while they travel that distance! Buying local and in season, as well as canning and freezing, can keep you supplied with chemical-free produce throughout the year. You'll need to set some priorities as to where you can cut back on hormones and antibiotics, however, although some major producers have now stopped using them. Read the packages! Then think about where you are getting the most? Meat, eggs, dairy? Focus on one and gradually change over the others later. Remember, clean eating is not all or nothing. Every step will bring its own benefits.

The next thing is to transition to eating smaller more frequent meals and snacks. This really does two things for you. When you eat every 3-5 hours, you avoid getting too hungry between meals. This makes it much easier to eat a smaller amount, particularly if you've increased your intake of complex carbohydrates like fruits and veggies. Many health experts recommend going no longer than 4-5 hours without a meal or snack for another reason. Frequent eating helps to prevent spikes in sugar levels, preventing energy highs and lows as well as keeping your hormone (insulin and glucagon) levels steady. Ensuring that you have both lean protein and complex carbs at each meal is also related to this balancing of the food-related hormones. Carbs cause the production of insulin, proteins glucagon. Too much of one or the other and you'll feel the effects later. After all, diabetes is a malfunction in insulin production that results in inadequate insulin levels. The problems inherent in this condition are well known. So, keeping these powerful hormones balanced through food consumption is important. Simply put, you'll feel better.

The final item is upping your water intake. We all know we should drink more water---not just liquid, water. Our bodies are mostly made of water, and they let us know when we haven't had enough. But most of us don't listen! Our bodies' everyday signs of dehydration are often mistakenly interpreted as hunger, fatigue, and even colds or allergies. Drinking an adequate amount of water daily may be the single healthiest thing you can do for yourself, regardless of what you eat. It's essential for weight loss as well, so keep that water bottle filled, with you---and drink it!

Chapter 4: Eating clean on a budget

The simplest way to eat cleaner is to buy organic products, but we all know that they generally cost more. Especially when feeding a family, this can seem like a major hurdle in eating clean. There are, however, some ways to make it work. It just takes some planning and organization. And, remember that this isn't all-or-nothing---make small changes and adaptations gradually but consistently and soon you'll be eating almost completely clean. You also need to identify and define what "clean eating" means to you. How much of this plan do you want to implement right now? Choose your main areas of concern and focus your efforts there. This is one way to keep your costs from suddenly skyrocketing.

Many web sites tell you to go through your cupboards, fridge, and freezer and ruthlessly discard or donate anything that's not clean. Then make a monster shopping trip to refill your kitchen with clean foods. Right, who can afford that? It's far more sensible to take a Saturday, check what you have on hand, and find the worst offenders in your pantry. Use them up and don't buy them again. Buy clean versions of those products instead. On each shopping trip, read labels and find clean (or clean-er) substitutes for the things you'd normally buy. Get whole-wheat pasta instead of regular; real maple syrup in place of artificial, quinoa not white rice. Gradual minor changes will be much easier on your pocketbook.

More and more companies are cleaning up their products, so take the time to read their labels, but watch out for added sugar or salt in canned goods. Explore the organic section. There are many prepackaged, frozen, and canned "clean" foods available there for reasonable prices. Again, read the labels---organic or "all natural" doesn't necessarily mean clean in the food business! The foodstuffs may be highly processed or have "natural" additives and still be organic!

Buy fresh or frozen when possible in place of canned. Every day there are more clean options in the freezer section, particularly fruits and veggies, including pre-chopped onions and other veggies for use in cooking. Again, be alert for added ingredients like sugar or salt. Your frozen blueberries should contain blueberries and that's it. But, if you have trouble using up fresh produce before it spoils, try frozen and you'll be able to use it all. You can also get out of season produce from the freezer aisle.

Buying clean meat, if you can't afford organic free-range, can be difficult. The local farmer's market (or butcher's shop) is a good place to start, or a store like Whole Foods. Even if you don't purchase there, they may be able to point you towards some small local farms. Be prepared to pay a bit more, however. Many people on a budget simply try to find the best compromise. Adding more meatless meals into your menu is one way to stretch the meat budget. That way, when you have meat it's high quality ... but you don't have it everyday. Another is to do some of the work yourself. Buy a whole chicken instead of pieces, and cut it up. It's usually much less expensive per pound! Boil the carcass and bones to make your own chicken broth for soups or cooking. Get the huge piece of beef (on sale) and divide it into smaller roasts at home, or get the butcher at the store to cut it up for you. And, use your freezer!

Eggs are fairly easy, but dairy in general is another tricky area for clean eaters. Many milk products, even organic, are homogenized and pasteurized, which are processes that change the milk. So does making it low fat or nonfat, which also involves added powdered dry milk to improve appearance. Milk that hasn't been processed in these ways is called "raw". It's hard to find raw milk, and it's actually illegal in many places, unless it comes from your own cow, since pasteurization is a process related to preventing the spread of tuberculosis. Raw milk from a healthy cow won't hurt you, and it definitely tastes better, just like fresh fish does. This is one of those areas where you definitely have to decide for yourself how far you want to go with "clean" eating, although many people choose dairy that avoids hormones and antibiotics and they don't worry so much about the processing. One note, however, is to always shred your own cheese---the pre-shredded has preservatives added!

While shopping smart can help you to begin to eat cleaner, planning and preparation are the way to integrate it into your daily life reasonably. Raising your own fruits and veggies is great, and do consider container gardening if you don't have much space. Growing fresh herbs on a windowsill is super easy! In season, go to the u-pick fields and stock up---it's a great family activity! The next step is keeping it for later use. Home canning has become popular again for exactly this reason, and many items can also be frozen very easily. With just a little research and some storage space, you can keep the season's bounty fresh for clean eating throughout the year.

Many of your favorite "convenience" items can be duplicated at home...and made clean. Again, it just takes planning and time. Shred your own cheese and package it up in small storage bags for use later. Make several batches of clean whole wheat (or white whole wheat) pizza dough and freeze them. If you have enough freezer space, go ahead and make up the pizzas. They'll be better than those store-bought frozen ones every time! Mix up your own salad dressings for the week. Make your own mayo. Love that taco seasoning mix? Combine the spices at home and bag it up in portions ready to use. Mix up those clean oatmeal cookies and freeze cookie size blobs for quick easy baking at a later time. The Internet can provide a surprising number of recipes for many of the items that you buy premixed or pre-packaged. Or you can read the ingredients off the package and experiment with the proportions on your own, leaving out the artificial stuff, of course. All these "make your own" items are not only "clean" but also taste better and cost less!

It also helps to get your kids involved, and not just in picking produce at local farms. Take them to the farmer's market with you. Challenge them to find unfamiliar foods they can learn about---they may want to try some! Involve them in menu planning, preparation, and cooking, and they'll be more willing to adjust to cleaner eating habits. They may even become eating clean Nazis, keeping *your* eating in line!

It is possible to eat clean without breaking the bank, but it takes some time and effort on your part. Start slowly, get the whole family involved, and be prepared to make a few decisions and compromises. Every change towards eating cleaner, no matter how small, is a step in a healthy direction.

Chapter 5: Eating clean on the go

With the hectic schedules many of us keep, it's often hard to avoid falling into bad eating habits. So how do you keep up with clean eating at school, work, the soccer game? Again planning and preparation are the keys. Setting aside a block of time to prep your food for the week saves twice the time later, even if you're not eating clean! Sometimes it's as simple as making a double-batch of lasagna and freezing half for a no-fuss meal next week, or mixing up and baking two casseroles at once for an eat-one-freeze-one special. Simmer up a triple pot of chili. These types of meals can also be saved as individual portions for quick microwavable lunches or dinners. Cooking several meals at once is also nice for your utility bill!

Pre-prep and package your vegetables for snacks, lunch boxes, or quick stir-fry's later on. Make ahead and freeze your own piecrust for quick hearty quiches or potpies. Go further, make and freeze whole fruit pies in season for baking months later! I remember my mother doing this. She'd get the "seconds" from local fruit farms---the fruit that was misshapen, too small or large, or had minor blemishes on the skin. They may not be as attractive for just eating but they're perfect for cooking!

Then she'd spend a day making and freezing pies. She saved a ton of money, and we enjoyed fresh baked peach or apple pies in the depths of winter.

And, definitely dust off that crock-pot! Slow cookers not only give you a hot meal without the fuss when you get home. They can help you prepare ahead of time for meals to come. Cook chicken overnight in the slow cooker, put the whole crock in the fridge in the morning, and slice or cube the chicken later. You can use it for dinner, freeze it, or both. You'll save time and money, and you'll still be able to eat clean! The same goes for soups and many other dishes. Your crock-pot can even help you with having a healthy "clean" breakfast, ready when you get up. Oatmeal is fantastic slow-cooked overnight! A slow-cooker cookbook can get you started---just substitute clean ingredients in the recipes. The possibilities are endless, and once you begin you'll quickly come up with your own.

Stock your pantry with nuts, pumpkin seeds, organic raisins, and other clean snack foods. Apart from snacking, substitute them for commercial potato chips in lunch boxes. There's a large variety of dried fruits in the organic section of the store that work very well for this, as do "clean" pretzels. Please don't forget eggs---a hard-boiled egg makes a healthy and protein-filled addition to either breakfast or lunch, and they can be prepared ahead of time and kept peeled in the refrigerator for quick packing or eating.

Fitting new eating habits into your busy lifestyle isn't hard if you take some time to plan for it. You may also find that the preparation time becomes a relaxing ritual for you. Dicing veggies or peeling apples doesn't require a lot of thought or attention, leaving your mind free to mull over other matters. The mechanical motions can also be very soothing. I know a couple who devote one Saturday morning a month to making their own "clean" bread. They've done it for years---mixing, kneading, talking, and just spending time together. They decompress from their high-pressured workweek and fill their freezer with great healthy bread at the same time! Definitely a win-win!

Chapter 6: Eating Clean for Weight Loss

If you want to shed some pounds, you'll need to follow some stricter guidelines. Eating clean won't automatically melt off the excess weight. It's not a magic bullet, no matter what some web sites may want you to believe. You'll need to focus on portion control, protein-carb balance, when you eat, and the actual nutrients in your food. Of course, adding extra physical activity helps as well!

Portion control is huge if you expect to lose weight. You know the dangers of "supersize me", but many people anymore are unaware of just what a normal size serving should be. It's been a long time since we've seen them! Even dinner plates have been supersized in the past 40 years! Standard everyday plates used to be 9 inches; it's hard nowadays to find any plates smaller than 10 ½ and many are 12 inches. That's a huge increase in surface area because it increases exponentially. An inch increase in diameter is much more than an inch more surface area. [Ask a math person and they can explain it to you.] What this means to portion control is that your normal sized serving looks inadequate and lost on your enormous plate! If you have what are called luncheon plates, usually 8 to 8½ inches, try using those. Your "normal" portions will fill your plate more pleasingly and it will look like more food. A psychological trick, yes, but it works! And you'll begin to scale back your eyes from the "supersize me" trap.

So what is a single serving? For meat and fish, it's generally the size of your palm, for veggies or starches, the size of your fist. Using this sort of "eyeball measure" helps you to see how much you're eating, even when you eat out. Most restaurants are really giving you double or triple servings. Eyeballing is also much quicker and easier than trying to weigh or measure everything. You can also picture your plate (not a jumbo plate!) as divided in 5 sections. You should have one of lean protein, one of healthy carb, and three of fruits and veggies.

Tosca Reno, who popularized clean eating, recommends that you write down your goals before you begin to help keep you focused---and keep them realistic! Starting your day with a good breakfast, such as oatmeal with fresh berries and a hard-boiled egg, will keep you feeling full all day, not just all morning. It has a long-term effect on both satiety and metabolism. Graze! Eat small amounts every 2-3 hours for optimal weight loss. This keeps your metabolism revved up, and it's a habit of naturally thin people.

To lose weight with clean eating, you also need to keep a closer watch on the nutrients in your food. Pair your proteins and carbs, and keep them in balance as much as possible. You'll need to limit your carbs to about 100-150g per day, and that's total carbs, which includes fruits and vegetables. You should also limit your intake of fruit due to its high sugar content since sugar of any kind makes you crave more sugar. But also avoid under-eating! It gives you less calories, true, but it slows your entire metabolism so you don't burn up the calories. Be aware of not just *how much* but also *what* you're eating.

We also need to return to dairy here for a minute. Apart from being *processed* foods, low-fat and nonfat dairy are not good for weight loss. Really. A 2005 study found that reduced-fat dairy products were actually *associated with weight gain*! Yikes!!! Whether this is due to the processing or to the addition of ingredients to compensate for the loss in taste, you're better off and will feel more satisfied with eating full fat dairy. I know this flies in the face of what you've been told for so long, but it appears to be true. Full fat plain yogurt with your own fruit added will help you shed pounds better than the reduced fat versions. If it's a little too tart for you, add some honey---and ditch that "healthy" spread in favor of real butter while you're at it.

Eat only until you're "contented" not "full". Eating more slowly helps you to learn to recognize when you've reached this point. Put away the rest for later; if eating out, bring the extra home. Naturally slim people do this all the time, so it's a habit that will help you not only lose weight but maintain that weight loss. "Half now, half later" is a weight control mantra that will serve you well. Learn to listen to your body.

Keeping your water intake levels high is also very important for weight loss. You should consume at least 2-3 liters a day. We need water more than food. I'm sure you've heard that three days without water will kill you, but it takes three weeks to starve! Dehydration is often mistaken for hunger, so adequate water is necessary to help keep your diet on track. It also assists in flushing toxins from your system on a regular basis. The first couple of days you'll need to visit the restroom more often, it's true, but your body will soon accept that it's finally getting adequate water and it'll adjust.

You'll also need to limit your caffeine intake since it's a natural diuretic causing you to lose water. This is a hard one for many people! If you're eating clean, you've already cut out the myriad soft drinks, energy drinks, and "health" drinks that contain caffeine because of their other ingredients. Try substituting some green or herbal teas (hot or chilled), or some lemonade made with a low calorie natural sweetener like honey or stevia. Don't, however, substitute them for your water. It's water, then other beverages!

It's also important to be aware of some items know as "diet-busters", healthy foods that can undo your weight loss plan and progress if you're not very careful with them. The first is granola, even clean homemade granola. It's very dense, and a serving size is actually very small, making it easy to eat too much. It's also heavily carb-laden and can increase your appetite for the entire day, so be wary. The next potential diet-buster is hummus. It's very popular right now, and, yes, it's very healthy. Hummus is also high fat so portions need to be very small. Again it's an easy item to overeat. Peanut butter…ditto.

The final two diet-busters have become ubiquitous, and, like the previous ones, they're sneaky. The first of them is smoothies. The readily available versions you'll find at the mall (or even health clubs) are usually supersized, giving you several servings in one container. They also often contain added sugar through using sugared fruit to improve the taste. This is a tricky weight-loss trap---"I only had a smoothie!" You may actually have downed three or four servings, along with many times your daily allotment of carbs! The same type of thing is true for diet-buster number five, wraps. The wrapper itself is dense and often large. Many are equivalent to three slices of bread! Their size also disguises just how much filling is rolled up in there. It can often be far more than a normal sandwich! To keep both of these items from deep-sixing your weight loss efforts, make your own. If you're buying them when you're out and about, greatly reduce the portion size by sharing with a friend or saving some for later. As with most of the diet-busters, the food itself is good for you but portion control is vital!

A final caveat for achieving your weight loss goals: avoid "diet" products. Very few protein bars, for instance, are clean and most contain quite a bit of sugar. They may have a good protein-carb balance but they're not using healthy carbs to do it. The same goes for diet shakes or drinks. You'll do better, feel more satisfied, and lose more weight if you stick with real food in controlled portions. After all, that's what clean eating is really all about, isn't it?

Conclusion

Thank you again for downloading this book!

I hope this book was able to help you to understand the how's and why's of eating cleaner and greener, and the impact that even just a few dietary changes can have on your life and our world.

The next step is to revise your grocery list, read a lot of labels ... then start eating cleaner!

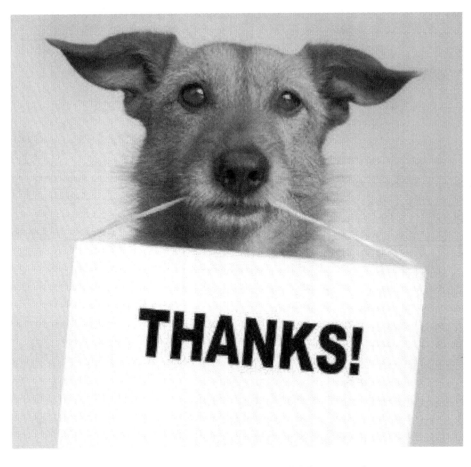

Finally, if you enjoyed this book, then I'd like to ask you for a favor, would you be kind enough to leave a review for this book on Amazon? It'd be greatly appreciated!

Click here to leave a review for this book on Amazon!

http://amzn.to/1qwaFgO

Thank you and good luck!

Check Out My Other Books

Below you'll find some of my other popular books that are popular on Amazon and Kindle as well. Simply click on the links below to check them out.

[Anti Inflammatory Diet: How to Fight Inflammation, Heart Disease and Chronic Pain just by Eating Delicious Food](#)

[Herbal Antibiotics & Antivirals: How to Cure Illness with Holistic, All Natural, Herbal Medicines and Remedies](#)

[Meditation for Beginners: Learn How to get a Healthy Mind, Body, and Spirit through Meditation](#)

[Mason Jar Meals: Quick and Easy Recipes for Meals on the Go, in a Jar](#)

If the links do not work, for whatever reason, you can simply search for these titles on the Amazon website to find them.

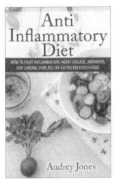 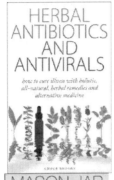 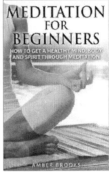

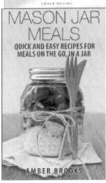

Don't Forget Your Free Bonus:
Get this FREE Report

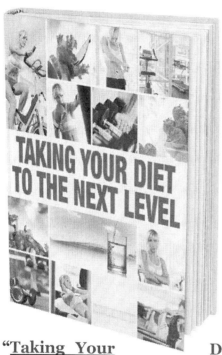

Do you want to lose weight, but nothing has worked long term? Do you have trouble changing your habits and end up falling back into the same unhealthy routine? Are you having trouble reaching the level of health and fitness success that you want to achieve? Well this Report is for you!!!

"Taking Your Diet to the Next Level" is an insightful report explaining why you aren't reaching the level of success that you want, and how to change that. It goes through each stage of dieting, weight loss and making healthy changes and provides strategies for how to break through those walls that are sopping you from achieving the diet, weight loss and fitness success that you deserve.

As a thank you, I want to give you this amazing report, completely free of charge, as my gift to you. There is no catch... it's really free, I promise. Just click the link below to download it now!

Click here to get it FREE!!

http://bit.ly/nextleveldiet

© Copyright 2014 - All rights reserved.

This document is geared towards providing exact and reliable information in regards to the topic and issue covered. The publication is sold with the idea that the publisher is not required to render accounting, officially permitted, or otherwise, qualified services. If advice is necessary, legal or professional, a practiced individual in the profession should be ordered.

- From a Declaration of Principles which was accepted and approved equally by a Committee of the American Bar Association and a Committee of Publishers and Associations.

In no way is it legal to reproduce, duplicate, or transmit any part of this document in either electronic means or in printed format. Recording of this publication is strictly prohibited and any storage of this document is not allowed unless with written permission from the publisher. All rights reserved.

The information provided herein is stated to be truthful and consistent, in that any liability, in terms of inattention or otherwise, by any usage or abuse of any policies, processes, or directions contained within is the solitary and utter responsibility of the recipient reader. Under no circumstances will any legal responsibility or blame be held against the publisher for any reparation, damages, or monetary loss due to the information herein, either directly or indirectly.

Respective authors own all copyrights not held by the publisher.

The information herein is offered for informational purposes solely, and is universal as so. The presentation of the information is without contract or any type of guarantee assurance.

The trademarks that are used are without any consent, and the publication of the trademark is without permission or backing by the trademark owner. All trademarks and brands within this book are for clarifying purposes only and are the owned by the owners themselves, not affiliated with this document.

Made in the USA
San Bernardino, CA
18 September 2016